THE DOCTOR'S QUOTATION BOOK

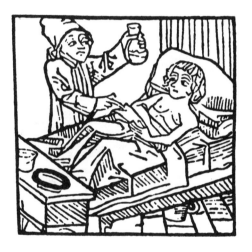

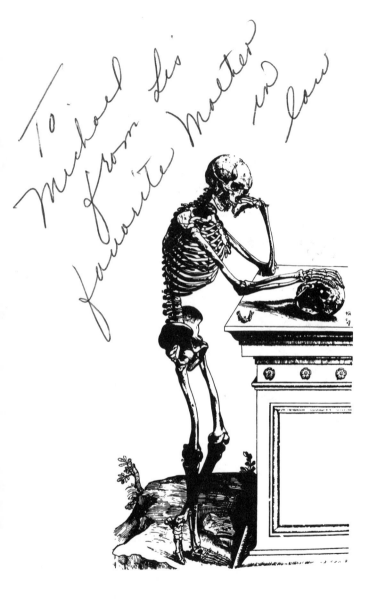

To Michael his
Michael his
from Master
favourite Master in
love

The
Doctor's
Quotation
Book

A Medical Miscellany

Edited by
DR ROBERT WILKINS

**BARNES
&NOBLE
BOOKS**
NEW YORK

This edition published by Marboro Books Corp.,
a division of Barnes & Noble, Inc.,
by arrangement with Robert Hale, Ltd.

1992 Barnes & Noble Books

ISBN 0-88029-881-2

Printed and bound in the United States of America

M 9 8 7 6 5 4 3 2

Preface

This is a little book which cannot hope to cover the sheer quantity and variety of medical writing. To attempt to be representative, much less comprehensive, would require a volume twenty times the size of this one. Consequently, at a very early stage in the selection process, I decided that the choice of quotations would be mine and mine alone, guided only by my own likes and dislikes, and my own personal preferences about what I considered memorable, insightful, ill-considered or humorous.

I have tried to admix aphorisms and anecdotes, and blend the one-liners with more detailed descriptions. I have also attempted to include lesser known authors: after all, it would be the easiest thing to fill this book with the wit and wisdom of Osler or Wendell Holmes, of Shakespeare's medical references, with the bons mots of the Hunter brothers or the cynicism which Shaw had to doctors and all things medical. If I have favoured any it is those doctors who found the expression of their genius in writing: John Keats, Conan Doyle and Somerset Maugham.

When the sources of some of the entries are not as complete as others, I have opted for inclusion rather than sacrifice.

The chances are high that you will only find a handful of your favourites, and that the majority of the medical quotations which *you consider indispensible are missing from this book. True to my initial resolve I make no apology, but hope that you will find some unfamiliar material to take your fancy. If you are still prone to grouse, you are welcome to write to the publisher to ask them to commission from me a longer work, which will give me the pleasure of delving again into the riches of the medical literature.*

One quote eluded me. From my student days I half remember a horticultural allusion to the appearance of the anus following haemorrhoidectomy: ' ... and if the op's a failure it looks like a dahlia'. But which flower did it resemble if all had gone according to plan?

ROBERT WILKINS
Paxton House, Reading

January 1991

Acknowledgements

I would like to thank the following people for helping me so much in the collection of material for this book. Enid Forsyth and Margaret Coleman at the Postgraduate Library, Royal Berkshire Hospital, Reading; Jinny Williams; Robert Williams; Kathleen Craig; Marie Crook; Miss E. Allen, Royal College of Surgeons; readers of the British Medical Journal and staff at the British Medical Association library.

Dedicated to
the late
Dr K. Bryn Thomas
whose collection of papers on
the history of medicine
gave me much of the material
included in this book

Physicians of all men are most happy; what good success soever they have, the world proclaimeth, and what faults they commit, the earth coverest.

FRANCIS QUARLES (1592–1644)
Nicocles

I don't want to be a doctor, and live by men's diseases; nor a minister to live by their sins; nor a lawyer to live by their quarrels. So I don't see anything left for me but to be an author.

NATHANIEL HAWTHORNE (1804–64)
in a remark to his mother

There are worse occupations in this world than feeling a woman's pulse.

LAURENCE STERNE (1713–68)
A Sentimental Journey

You advise me not to pursue two hares at a time and to abandon the practice of medicine ... I feel more contented and more satisfied when I realize that I have two professions, not one. Medicine is my lawful wife and literature my mistress. When I grow weary of one, I pass the night with the other ... neither of them suffers because of my infidelity.

ANTON CHEKHOV (1860–1904)
letter, 11 October 1889

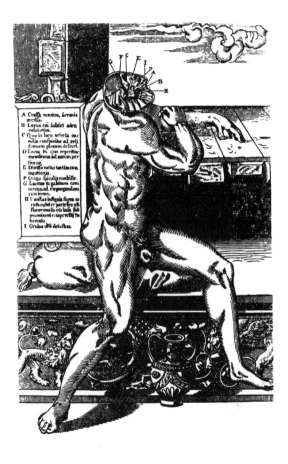

By Charles Estienne (1545)

Physicians and politicians resemble one another in this respect, that some defend the constitution and others destroy it.

> ANON
> From *Acton or the Circle of Life* (nineteenth century)

Physicians, like beer, are best when they are old.

> THOMAS FULLER (1608–61)
> *The Holy State and the Profane State*

Never forget that it is not a pneumonia, but a pneumonic man who is your patient.

> SIR WILLIAM GULL (1816–90)

First the patient, second the patient, third the patient, fourth the patient, fifth the patient, and then maybe comes science.

> BELA SCHICK (1877–1967)
> *Aphorisms and Facetiae of Bela Schick*

Physician, heal thyself.

> ST LUKE 4:23

I know of nothing more laughable than a doctor who does not die of old age.

> VOLTAIRE (1694–1778)
> in a letter to Charles Augustin Feriol

That physician will hardly be thought very careful of the health of others who neglects his own.

> GALEN
> *Of Protecting the Health*

We entrust ... our bodies to physicians, who, to a man, loathe medicine and refuse to take physics.
FRANÇOIS RABELAIS (?1494–1553)
Pantagruel

No doctor takes pleasure in the health even of his friends.
MICHEL DE MONTAIGNE (1533–92)
Essays

There are only two sorts of doctors: those who practise with their brains, and those who practise with their tongues.
SIR WILLIAM OSLER (1849–1919)
Counsels and Ideas

There are only two classes of mankind in the world – doctors and patients.
RUDYARD KIPLING (1865–1936)
speaking to medical students in 1908

Let no one suppose that the words doctor and patient can disguise from the parties the fact that they are employer and employee.
GEORGE BERNARD SHAW (1856–1950)
The Doctor's Dilemma

With us ther was a Doctour of Phisyk,
In al this world ne was ther noon hym lik,
To speke of physik and of surgerye,
For he was grounded in astronomye ...

He knew the cause of everich maladye,
Were it of hoot, or coold, or moyste, or drye,
And where they engendred, and of what humour;
He was a verray parfit praktisour.
GEOFFREY CHAUCER (*c.* 1345–1400)
The Canterbury Tales

When people's ill, they comes to I,
I physics, bleeds, and sweats 'em;
Sometimes they live, sometimes they die,
What's that to I? I let's 'em.
JOHN LETTSOM (1744–1815)
on himself

The King employs three doctors daily;
Willis, Heberden and Baillie;
All extremely clever men,
Baillie, Willis, Heberden;
But doubtful which most sure to kill is
Baillie, Heberden or Willis.
ANON
contemporary verse about the royal physicians of
George III

I'll do what Mead and Cheselden advise
To keep these limbs and to preserve these eyes.
ALEXANDER POPE (1688–1744)
immortalizing two eighteenth-century medical men.
(Cheselden once extracted a bladder stone in
fifty-four seconds.)

This leach Arbuthnot was yclept,
Who many a night not once had slept,
But watch'd our gracious Sovereign still;
For who could rest when she was ill?
Oh, mayst thou henceforth sweetly sleep.
Shear, swains, oh shear your softest sheep
To swell his couch; for well I ween,
He saved the Realm who saved the Queen.
  JOHN GAY (1685–1732)
  tribute to John Arbuthnott (1667–1735), physician
  to Queen Anne

'Do you remember the story they tell of Abernethy?'

'No; hang Abernethy!'

'To be sure! Hang him and welcome. But, once upon a time, a certain rich miser conceived the design of spunging upon this Abernethy for a medical opinion. Getting up, for this purpose, an ordinary conversation in a private company, he insinuated his case to the physician as that of an imaginery individual.

"We will suppose," said the miser, "that his symptoms are such and such; now, doctor, what would *you* have directed him to take?"

"Take!" said Abernethy, "why, take *advice*, to be sure." '
  EDGAR ALLAN POE (1809–49)
  The Purloined Letter

Since the last number of this Journal was published, that strange compound of talent and eccentricity, of enlightened observation and hobby-horsical empiricism, of

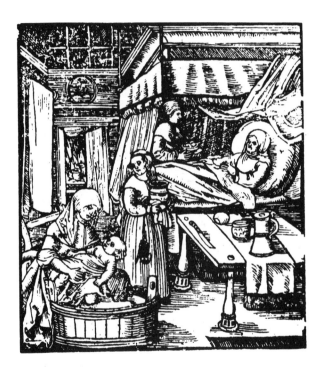

Childbirth by Rösslin (1541)

goodness of heart and rudeness of manner, of amiable feeling and irritable temper, has paid the debt of Nature.

ANON

the beginning of John Abernethy's obituary (1764–1831) in *The Medico-Chirurgical Review*, 1831

I have been a humble hum-drum teacher of anatomy for the last thirty years, and for the last five and twenty have not practised at all. My principal appearances, nowadays, are as an ornamental listener – not certainly from any charm of personal presence but because in this raw country anybody who has written a story or two or a few verses becomes thereby a stage-property for exhibition on public occasions.

OLIVER WENDELL HOLMES (1809–94)

declining an invitation to attend an international medical congress in 1876

After what seemed quite a long time, he put down his papers and said impatiently: 'I don't know why they are making such a fuss. There's nothing wrong with me.' He picked up his papers and resumed his reading. At last he pushed the bed-rest away and, throwing back the bed clothes said abruptly: 'I suffer from dyspepsia, and this is the treatment.' With that he proceeded to demonstrate to me some breathing exercises. His big white belly was moving up and down when there was a knock on the door, and the PM grabbed at the sheet as Mrs Hill came into the room.

LORD MORAN (1882–1977)

on his first consultation with Winston Churchill, 1940

Give me a doctor partridge-plump,
Short in the leg and broad in the rump,
An endomorph with gentle hands
Who'll never make absurd demands
That I abandon all my vices
Nor pull a long face in a crisis,
But with a twinkle in his eye
Will tell me that I have to die.
    W.H. AUDEN (1907–73)
    Nones

Never believe what a patient tells you his doctor said.
    SIR WILLIAM JENNER (1815–98)

A family doctor's life is awash with contrast: on the one hand he is feted and revered as a pillar of the community, often an elected mason and sometimes president of the cricket team; on the other hand he is at the beck and call of the lowliest of his patients who would demand his presence in the middle of the night to attend to a life-threatening runny nose.
    AN ANONYMOUS GENERAL PRACTITIONER

The world ... has long ago decided that you have no working hours that anyone is bound to respect, and nothing except extreme bodily illness will excuse you in its eyes from refusing to help a man who thinks he may need your help at any hour of the day or night. Nobody will care whether you are in your bed or in your bath, on your holiday or at the theatre.
    RUDYARD KIPLING (1865–1936)
    talking to medical students in 1908

There is no harder worker in all Scotland, and none more poorly requited, than the village doctor, unless perhaps it be his horse.

SIR WALTER SCOTT (1771–1832)
description of Dr Gideon Gray in *The Surgeon's Daughter*, and his two horses Pestle and Mortar

A sort of wonderful nondescript creature on two legs, something between a man and an Angel.

JANE AUSTEN (1775–1817)
description of her friend, Dr Charles Thomas Haden (1786–1824)

At the sight of that terrible charnel house – the fragments of limbs, the grinning heads and gaping skulls, the bloody quagmire underfoot and the atrocious smell it gave off, the swarms of sparrows wrangling over scraps of lungs, the rats in the corners gnawing the bleeding vertebrae – such a feeling of revulsion possessed me that I leapt through the window of the dissecting room and fled for home as though Death and all his hideous train were at my heels.

The objects which before had filled me with extreme horror had absolutely no effect on me now. I felt nothing but a cold distaste; I was already as hardened to the scene as any seasoned medical student. The crisis was past. I found I was actually enjoying groping about in a poor fellow's chest and feeding the winged inhabitants of that delightful place their ration of lung ... tossing a shoulder-blade to a great rat who was staring at me with famished eyes.

HECTOR BERLIOZ (1803–69)
Memoirs
about his time as a medical student in the early 1820s

Mr Bob Sawyer, who was habited in a coarse blue coat, which, without being either a great coat or a surtout, partook of the nature and qualities of both, had about him that sort of slovenly smartness, and swaggering gait, which is peculiar to young gentlemen who smoke in the streets by day, shout and scream in the same by night, call waiters by their christian names, and do various other acts and deeds of a facetious description. He wore a pair of plaid trousers and a large double-breasted waistcoat ... He eschewed gloves, and looked, upon the whole, something like a dissipated Robinson Crusoe.

> CHARLES DICKENS (1812–70)
> *The Pickwick Papers*
> description of a medical student

The pleasures and amusements [of medical students in the 1830s] then were coarser. There was much more drinking ... Cursing and swearing were common in ordinary talk ... Impurity of life and conversation were scarcely thought disgraceful or worth concealing ... But let me repeat, the students of that time were only living and talking after the ordinary manner of the day.

> SIR JAMES PAGET (1814–99)
> addressing the Abernethian Society, 1885

I was falling sick; but you came at once to me,
O Symmachus, attended by your hundred pupils.
A hundred hands frozen by the North Wind have pawed me:
O Symmachus, I had no fever then, but now I have.

> MARTIAL (*c.* 40–*c.* 104 AD)
> to his doctor, Symmachus

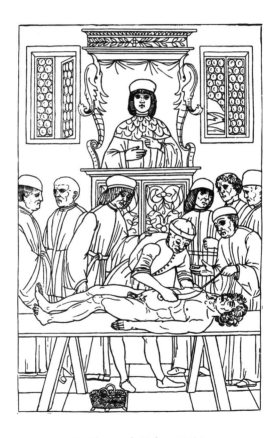

By Johannes de Ketham (1491)

The physician must have a worthy appearance; he should look healthy and be well-nourished, appropriate to his physique; for most people are of the opinion that those physicians who are not tidy in their own persons cannot look after others well. Further, he must look to the cleanliness of his person; he must wear decent clothes and use perfumes with harmless smells.

    HIPPOCRATES

His neckerchief and shirt-frill were ever of the whitest; his clothes were of the blackest and sleekest; his gold watch chain of the heaviest and his seals of the largest. His boots, which were always of the brightest, creaked as he walked ... and he had a peculiar way of smacking his lips and saying 'Ah' at intervals while patients detailed their symptoms, which inspired great confidence.

    CHARLES DICKENS (1812–70)
    Martin Chuzzlewit
    description of Dr Jobling, general practitioner

Each examiner was more or less a surgical celebrity, almost necessarily possessing some peculiarity in his experience or some singularity of view, I will not say crotchet; a fact which occasionally gave rise to a series of questions, unfortunate for a student who, well grounded in the principles and in the general practice of his art, might have no acquaintance with the peculiarities in question, and thus might fail to give the answers expected by the examiners.

    SIR HENRY THOMPSON (1820–1904)
    Charley Kingston's Aunt, 1885
    one of the most eminent surgeons of his day on the
    traumas of the membership examination

Examiner, utilizing information he had read the previous evening: 'Tell me, which animal does not have a gall bladder?'
Candidate: 'The kangaroo, sir.'
Examiner, taken aback: 'What about the horse?'
Candidate: 'What about the kangaroo?'

> VIVA ANECDOTE
> unattributable, and almost certainly apocryphal

Then at my second table Hodgson examined me. He was very jolly, began joking me about my name, asked me if I was a descendant of Sir Isaac ... told me the best life of Sir Isaac was in a small book by King, recommended me to get it. Then asked me if I knew what he died of; I thought apoplexy, told me stone.

> ISAAC NEWTON (1838–1922)
> on his MRCS examination in 1859. He passed

O, O, O to touch and feel a girl's vagina and hymen.

> TRADITIONAL
> medical student's mnemonic for the names of the twelve cranial nerves

A young man, in whose air and countenance appeared all the uncouth gravity and supercilious self-conceit of a physician hot from his studies.

> TOBIAS SMOLLETT (1721–71)
> *The Adventures of Peregrine Pickle*

In illness the physician is a father; in convalescence, a friend; when health is restored, he is a guardian.

> BRAHMANIC SAYING

Fifty years ago the successful doctor was said to need three things: a top hat to give him Authority, a paunch to give him Dignity, and piles to give him an Anxious Expression.

    ANONYMOUS CONTRIBUTOR TO THE *LANCET*, 1951

Doctors are men who prescribe medicine of which they know little to cure diseases of which they know less in human beings of which they know nothing.

    VOLTAIRE (1694–1778)

No families take so little medicine as those of doctors, except those of apothecaries.

    OLIVER WENDELL HOLMES (1809–94)
    Medical Essays

Medical men don't know the drugs they use, nor their prices.

    ROGER BACON (?1214–94)
    De Erroribus Medicorum

    Three shapes a doctor wears. At first we hail
    The angel; then the god, if he prevail.
    Last, when the cure complete, he asks his fee,
    A hideous demon he appears to be.

    ANONYMOUS LATIN POEM
    quoted by W.F.H. King in *Classical Foreign Quotations*

If a doctor has treated a gentleman for a severe wound with a bronze lancet and has cured him, or if he has opened with a bronze lancet an abscess of the eye of a gentleman and has

healed the man's eye, he shall accept ten shekels of silver
… If a doctor has treated a gentleman with a bronze lancet
for a severe wound and has caused him to die, or if he has
opened with a bronze lancet an abscess of the eye of a
gentleman and has caused the loss of the eye, the doctor's
hands shall be cut off.

THE CODE OF KING HAMMURABI (1728–1686 BC)
Babylonian king

The chief defect of Henry King
Was chewing little bits of string.
At last he swallowed some which tied
Itself in ugly Knots inside.
Physicians of the Utmost Fame
Were called at once; but when they came
They answered, as they took their Fees,
'There is no cure for this disease.'

HILAIRE BELLOC (1870–1953)
Cautionary Tales for Children

They [doctors], on the whole, desire to cure the sick; and –
if they are good doctors and the choice were fairly put to
them – would rather cure their patient and lose their fee,
than kill him and get it.

JOHN RUSKIN (1819–1900)
The Crown of Wild Olive

Crito, I owe a cock to Aesculapius. Will you remember to
pay the debt?

SOCRATES
last words

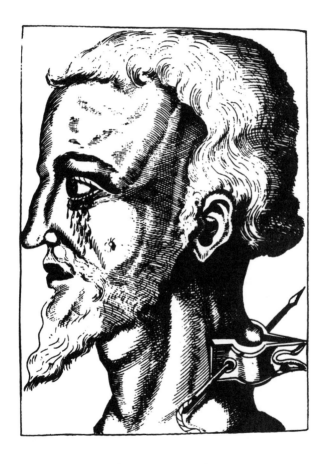

Use of seton to cure a running eye

When men a dangerous disease did 'scape
Of old, they gave a cock to Aesculape.
Let me give two, that doubly am got free
From my disease's danger, and from thee.
> BEN JOHNSON (1573–1637)
> *'To Dr Empirick'*

A fashionable surgeon like a pelican can be recognized by the size of his bill.
> J. CHALMERS DA COSTA (1863–1933)
> *The Trials and Triumphs of the Surgeon*

A physician who heals for nothing is worth nothing.
> THE TALMUD

That little dirty village quack sent in his bill. Never paid money with more reluctance.
> LADY ELEANOR BUTLER (1745–1829)
> diary entry for 4 October 1788

Dear Brother,
The bearer is very desirous of having your opinion … He has no money, and you don't want any, so that you are well met.

Ever yours.
John Hunter
> JOHN HUNTER (1728–93)
> letter to his brother William

He [Dr James Ripley] pulled up his fifty guinea chestnut mare and took a look at it [a brass plate]. 'Verrinder Smith MD' was printed across it in very neat small lettering … He

... consulted the current medical directory. By it he learned that Dr Verrinder Smith was the holder of superb degrees, that he had studied with distinction at Edinburgh, Paris, Berlin and Vienna, and finally that he had been awarded a gold medal at the Lee Hopkins scholarship for original research ...

He drove over the next day and called upon Dr Verrinder Smith ... Turning round, he found himself facing a little woman, whose plain, palish face was remarkable only for a pair of shrewd, humorous eyes ...

'How do you do, Dr Ripley?' said she.

'How do you do, madam?' returned the visitor. 'Your husband is perhaps out?'

'I am not married,' she said simply.

'Oh, I beg your pardon! I meant the doctor – Dr Verrinder Smith.'

'I am Dr Verrinder Smith.'

Dr Ripley was so surprised that he dropped his hat and forgot to pick it up again ... He could not recall any Biblical injunction that the man should remain ever the doctor and the woman the nurse, and yet he felt as if a blasphemy had been committed.

> SIR ARTHUR CONAN DOYLE (1859–1930)
> *The Doctors of Hoyland*

Day before yesterday, for the first time since its foundation several centuries ago, a petticoat might be seen in the august amphitheatre of the *Ecole de Médecine*. That petticoat enrobed the form of your most obedient servant and dutiful daughter!

> MARY PUTNAM JACOBI (1842–1906)
> letter to her mother, 1868

An examiner, no lover of females, thrust a femur into her hand.

'How many of those have you got?' he demanded.

'Five.'

'How do you come to that conclusion?' he asked contemptuously.

'I have two of my own, the one in my hand, and the two of my unborn child.'

> ANONYMOUS ANECDOTE
> I trust she passed

Let Surgeon MacArdle confirm you in Hope
A jockey fell off and his neck it was broke
He lifted him up like a fine honest man
And he said, 'He is dead, but I'll do all I can.'

> OLIVER ST JOHN GOGARTY (1878–1957)
> about an ENT surgeon colleague

These articles being removed [coat and neckerchief], he snatched off his wig, placing it on the gun-deck capstan; then took out his set of false teeth, and placed it by the side of the wig; and, lastly, putting his forefinger to the inner angle of his blind eye, spirited out the glass optic with professional dexterity, and deposited that, also, next to the wig and false teeth. Thus divested of nearly all inorganic appurtenances, what was left of the Surgeon slightly shook itself, to see whether anything more could be spared to advantage.

> HERMAN MELVILLE (1819–91)
> *White Jacket*
> describing how Cadwallader Cuticle MD, Surgeon of
> the Fleet, prepared to perform an on-board
> amputation

A surgeon should be young, a physician old.
    FRENCH PROVERB

Dogged by ill-health 'Billy' Lucas had never been fit enough to study anatomy in the unhealthy dissecting-rooms of the day; but the influence of a successful father proved stronger than this handicap and in 1799 he succeeded to the parental position as surgeon in the hospital. Here he began a career of butchery ... He put students off surgery, not as has been suggested because he was dull, but because he was dangerous; the person most to appreciate the danger was his own dresser, left to clear up the mess he had made.
    ROBERT GITTINGS (1911–   )
    The dresser was John Keats

The glory of surgeons is like that of actors which lasts only for their own lifetime and can no longer be appreciated once they have passed away. Actors and surgeons ... are all heroes of the moment.
    HONORÉ DE BALZAC (1799–1850)
    The Human Comedy

Wonderful cures he had done, O yes,
but they said too of him
He was happier using the knife than in
trying to save the limb,
And that I can well believe, for he
look'd so coarse and so red,
I could think he was one of those
who would break their jests on the dead.
    ALFRED, LORD TENNYSON (1809–92)
    'In the Children's Hospital'

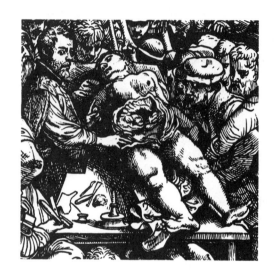

Vesalius giving an anatomy lecture

Time has produced a most absurd custom of measuring the motion of a surgeon's hand as jockeys do that of the feet of a horse, viz., by a stop-watch, a practice which, though it may have been encouraged by the operators themselves, must have been productive of most mischievous consequences.

PERCIVALL POTT (1714–88)
Observations on the Fistula Lachrymalis, 1775

Now it cannot be too often repeated that when an operation is once performed, nobody can ever prove that it was unnecessary. If I refuse to allow my leg to be amputated, its mortification and my death may prove that I was wrong; but if I let the leg go, nobody can ever prove that it would not have mortified had I been obstinate. Operation is therefore the safe side for the surgeon as well as the lucrative side.

GEORGE BERNARD SHAW (1856–1950)
The Doctor's Dilemma

There is no person, let his situation in life be what it may, whom, if I were disposed to dissect, I could not obtain.

SIR ASTLEY COOPER (1768–1841)
surgeon to royalty, explaining to the House of
Commons Committee how he acquired bodies for
anatomical dissection

Ask the opinion of a dozen medical men upon the novel in which the doctor is best described, and the majority will say *Middlemarch*.

SIR WILLIAM OSLER (1849–1919)

31

Since I saw you, a medical man at Ealing has written to me to express his regret that I have 'blotted' the correctness of my representation of medical subjects, by speaking of Lydgate's 'bright dilated eyes' in such a connection as to imply that an opiate would have the effect of dilating the pupil. It is a piece of contemptible forgetfulness in me, that when I wrote these passages I had not present in my mind the fact which I had read again and again – that one of the effects of opium is to contract the pupil ... And what I wish to ask of your goodness now is, to tell me whether you think the matter grave enough to urge my cancelling the two stereotype plates (certainly no great affair) before any more copies are struck off.

GEORGE ELIOT (1819–80)
writing to her friend Sir James Paget about
Middlemarch

He went to study in Paris with the determination that when he came home again he would settle in some provincial town as a general practitioner, and resist the irrational severance between medical and surgical knowledge in the interests of his own scientific pursuits, as well as of the general advance: he would keep away from the range of London intrigues, jealousies, and social truckling, and win celebrity, however slowly, as Jenner had done, by the independent value of his work.

GEORGE ELIOT (1819-80)
Middlemarch
describing Dr Lydgate's early optimism

Shall I, who even in the morning of my days, sought the lowly and sequestered paths of life, the valley, and not the mountain; shall I, now my evening is fast approaching, hold myself up as an object for fortune and for fame? Admitting it as a certainty that I obtain both, what stock should I add to my little fund of happiness? My fortune ... is sufficient to gratify my wishes; ... And as for fame, what is it? a gilded butt, forever pierced with the arrows of malignancy.

> EDWARD JENNER (1749–1823)
> discoverer of smallpox vaccination, on being enticed
> from his beloved Gloucestershire to take up practice
> in London

And whatsoever I shall see or hear in the course of my profession, as well as outside my profession in my intercourse with men, if it be what should not be published abroad, I will never divulge, holding such things to be holy secrets.

> PART OF THE HIPPOCRATIC OATH
> between 5th century BC and 1st century AD

Most people have a furious itch to talk about themselves and are restrained only by the disinclination of others to listen. Reserve is an artificial quality that is developed in most of us as the result of innumerable rebuffs. The doctor is discreet. It is his business to listen and no details are too intimate for his ears.

> W. SOMERSET MAUGHAM (1874–1965)
> *The Summing Up*

I deny the lawfulness of telling a lie to a sick man for fear of alarming him. You have no business with consequences; you are to tell the truth. Besides, you are not sure what effect your telling him that he is in danger may have. It may

bring his distemper to a crisis, and that may cure him. Of all lying, I have the greatest abhorrence of this, because I believe it has frequently been practised on myself.
    SAMUEL JOHNSON (1709–84)

Before you tell the 'truth' to the patient, be sure you know the 'truth', and that the patient wants to hear it.
    RICHARD CLARKE CABOT (1868–1939)
    Journal of Chronic Diseases, 1963

Most patients assume
dying is something they do,
not their physician,
that white-coated sage,
never to be imagined
naked or married.
    W.H. AUDEN (1907–73)
    'In Memoriam David Protetch, MD'

A point that stands out prominently in my experience is the frequency of the disease [angina pectoris] in our profession. For the same reason doubtless that Sydenham gives for the incidence of gout 'more wise men than fools are afflicted', angina may almost be called 'morbus medicorum'.
    SIR WILLIAM OSLER (1849–1919), 1897

My life is in the hands of any fool who cares to upset me.
    JOHN HUNTER (1728–93)
    Scottish surgeon, and sufferer from angina, who died
    of a heart attack following a dispute with a colleague

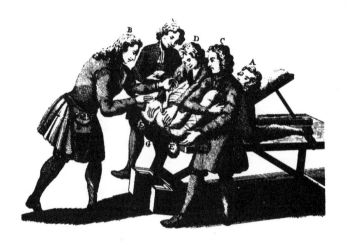

Patient held for operation to remove bladder stone

It was a French physician, quite naturally, who first described the disease known as cirrhosis of the liver. His name, René Théophile Hyacinthe Laënnec. This fastidious gentleman was the very same whose aversion to applying his naked ear to the perfumed but unbathed bosoms of his patients inspired him to invent the stethoscope ... The entire medical world continues to pay homage to Laënnec for his gift of space interpersonal.

> RICHARD SELZER (1928–)
> *Mortal Lessons*

In 1816, I was consulted by a young woman labouring under the general symptoms of diseased heart and in whose case percussion and the application of the hand were of little avail on account of the great degree of fatness ... I happened to recollect a simple and well-known fact in acoustics ... The fact I allude to is the great distinctness with which we can hear the scratch of a pin at one end of a piece of wood on applying our ear to the other. Immediately, on this suggestion, I rolled a quire of paper into a kind of cylinder and applied one end of it to the region of the heart and the other to my ear and was not a little surprised and pleased to find that I could thereby perceive the action of the heart in a manner much more clear and distinct than I had ever been able to do by the immediate application of the ear.

> RENÉ LAËNNEC (1781–1826)

The deplorable method of instruction which is used today demands that one person – generally a surgeon or barber – should carry out the dissection of the human body, while the lecturer reads a description of the different parts of the body derived from books ... Those who are actually performing the dissection are so ignorant that they are in fact not in a position to demonstrate to the students the parts which they are preparing, or to explain them, and as the professor never touches the body and as the dissector does not know the Latin names and therefore cannot follow the lecture in sequence, each goes his own way ... in the confusion the student learns less than a butcher could teach the professor.

> ANDREAS VESALIUS (1515–64)
> *De Humani Corporis Fabrica*

Madame, I have beneath my feet at this moment a foot-stool which I have never seen, but I turn it over with my feet and find it has four legs of wood and a soft top, and it is square.

> SIR HENRY THOMPSON (1820–1904)
> describing, over dinner, to the Empress Eugénie how he had gauged the size of Napoleon III's bladder stone

That is all very fine, but it won't do – anatomy, botany. Nonsense, Sir! I know an old woman in Covent Garden who understands botany better, and as for anatomy, my butcher can dissect a joint full as well. No, young man, all this is stuff: you must go to the bedside, it is there alone you can learn disease.

> THOMAS SYDENHAM (1624–89)
> Cromwellian physician, who was dubbed 'the English Hippocrates'

The road to medical knowledge is through the pathological museum, and not through an apothecary's shop.

> SIR WILLIAM GULL (1816–90)

I believe, indeed, that fifty years ago the admission of young ladies to be nurses in this [St Bartholomew's] or any similar hospital could not have been seriously proposed. It would have been called indecent, audacious, unprincipled, and I know not what besides; and the notion of their being associated with medical students would have been deemed utterly vile; nothing but vile mischief would have been foretold of it.

> SIR JAMES PAGET (1814–99)
> views on nursing in the 1830s

Lectured at by committees, preached at by chaplains, scowled on by treasurers and stewards, scolded by matrons, sworn at by surgeons, bullied by [surgical] dressers, grumbled at and abused by patients, insulted if old and ill-favored, talked flippantly to if middle-aged and good humoured, seduced if young – they are what any woman would be under the same circumstances.

> THE TIMES, 1857
> description of pre-Nightingale nurses

Nor bring to watch me cease to live
Some Doctor, full of phrase and fame
To shake his sapient head and give
The ill he can not cure – a name.

> MATTHEW ARNOLD (1822–88)
> 'A Wish'

When a disease is named after some author, it is very likely that we don't know much about it.

> AUGUST BIER (1861–1949)

Many years ago, I saw a fundus oculi with patches of black pigment on it scattered all over the field, so I asked an ophthalmic consultant to give me his opinion. He wrote in the notes: 'This is retinitis pigmentosa. It might be part of the Laurence Moon Biedl syndrome. Is there any evidence of polydactyly?' Surely, to refer a patient back to a physician to have the number of his fingers counted argues a degree of specialisation which has altogether obliterated common sense.

> RICHARD ASHER (1912–69)
> *Richard Asher Talking Sense*, 1973

Caution and fear are different things: where any good can be done, it ought to be attempted by every practical and justifiable means; but when no good is reasonably to be expected, there is no warrent for doing anything.

> PERCIVALL POTT (1714–88)
> *Injuries of the Head*, 1775

The mistakes made by doctors are innumerable. They err habitually on the side of optimism as to treatment, of pessimism as to the outcome. 'Wine? In moderation, it can do you no harm, it's always a tonic. Sexual enjoyment? After all it's a natural function. But you mustn't overdo it, you understand. Excess in anything is wrong.' At once, what a temptation to the patient to renounce those two life-givers, water and chastity!

> MARCEL PROUST (1871–1922)
> *Remembrance of Times Past*, Vol. 2

Faith, sir, our cat is lately recovered of a fall she had from the top of the house into the street, and was three days without either eating or moving foot or paw; but 'tis very

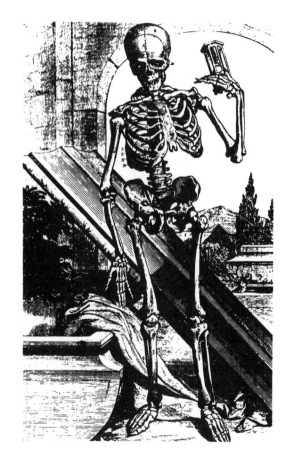

By Godfried Bidloo (1685)

lucky for her that there are no cat-doctors, for 'twould have
been over with her, and they would not have failed purging
her and bleeding her.
>MOLIÈRE (1622–73)
>*L'Amour Médecin*

Every day, and in every way, I am getting better and better.
>EMIL COUÉ (1857–1926)
>*Auto-Suggestion*, 1922

It is well to be up before daybreak, for such habits
contribute to health, wealth and wisdom.
>ARISTOTLE (384–322 BC)

Early to rise and early to bed
Makes a male healthy, wealthy and dead.
>JAMES THURBER (1894–1961)

People who are always taking care of their health are like
misers, who are hoarding up a treasure which they have
never spirit enough to enjoy.
>LAURENCE STERNE (1713–68)

There are two things in life that a sage must preserve at
every sacrifice, the coats of his stomach and the enamel of
his teeth. Some evils admit of consolations, but there are
no comforters for dyspepsia and the toothache.
>HENRY LYTTON BULWER, (1801–72)

To get back my youth I would do anything in the world,
except take exercise, get up early or be respectable.
>OSCAR WILDE (1854–1900)
>*The Picture of Dorian Gray*

The antipathy I have for their [doctors'] art is hereditary with me. My father lived seventy-four years, my grandfather sixty-nine, my great-grandfather nearly eighty, without having tasted any sort of medicine.

    MICHEL DE MONTAIGNE (1533–92)
    Essays

He who immerses himself in sexual intercourse will be assailed by premature ageing, his strength will wane, his eyes will weaken, and a bad odour will emit from his mouth and his armpits, his teeth will fall out and many other maladies will afflict him.

    MAIMONIDES (1135–1204)
    Mishreh Torah

There was an old fellow named Hewing,
Whose heart stopped while he was screwing;
He gasped: 'Really, Miss,
Don't feel bad about this –
There's nothing I'd rather die doing.'

    ANON

A man of sixty has spent twenty years in bed and over three years eating.

    ARNOLD BENNETT (1867–1931)

Persons who are naturally very fat are apt to die earlier than those who are slender.

    HIPPOCRATES
    Aphorisms

Never be afraid of open windows. People don't catch cold in bed. This is a popular fallacy. With proper bed-clothes and hot bottles you can always keep a patient warm in bed and well ventilate him at the same time ... I know an intelligent humane house surgeon who makes a practice of keeping the ward windows open. The physicians and surgeons invariably close them while going their rounds; and the house surgeon very properly as invariably opens them whenever the doctors have turned their backs.

FLORENCE NIGHTINGALE (1820–1910)
Notes on Nursing, 1859

A custome lothsome to the eye, hateful to the Nose, harmefull to the braine, dangerous to the Lungs, and the blacke stinking fume thereof, neerest resembling the horrible Stigian smoke of the pit that is bottomlesse.

JAMES I (1566–1625)
A Counter-Blaste to Tobacco

I have made it a rule never to smoke more than one cigar at a time.

MARK TWAIN (1835–1910)

If you want to keep a dead man, put him in whisky; if you want to kill a live man put whisky in him.

THOMAS GUTHRIE (1803–73)
Scottish divine and social reformer

We were so happy till Father drank rum,
Then all our sorrow and trouble begun;
Mother grew paler, and wept ev'ry day,
Baby and I were too hungry to play.
Slowly they faded, and one Summer's night

Found their dear faces all silent and white;
Then with big tears slowly dropping, I said:
'Father's a Drunkard, and Mother is dead!'
>   WRITTEN BY 'STELLA',
>   MUSIC BY MRS. E. A. PARKHURST

The secret of my abundant health is that whenever the
impulse to exercise comes over me, I lie down until it passes
away.
>   ANON
>   quoted by J. P. McEvoy in *American Mercury*,
>   December 1938

My eighteen-mile walk to Hastings is becoming quite a
common thing now; not long ago I walked there on a
Thursday and again on the *Saturday!* I hardly feel tired now
when I get there.
>   LEWIS CARROLL (1832–98)
>   letter to his sister Louisa, 1897

I get my exercise acting as a pallbearer to my friends who
exercise.
>   CHAUNCEY DEPEW (1834–1928)
>   American politician

As concerning the brynging up, nourishment and gevyng
of suckle to the chylde, it shal be beste that the mother
geve her chylde sucke her selfe, for the mothers milke is
more conveniente and agreeable to the Infant then any
other woman's ...
>   THOMAS RAYNALDE
>   *The Byrthe of Mankynde*, 1540

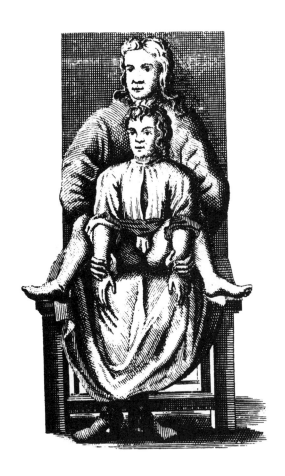

A child in position for removal of bladder stone

But, alas! too often for the want of due attention to its training, the tender plant is injured, and the charming blossoms of virtue and happiness are blighted.

JAMES PARKINSON (1755–1824)
Observations on the excessive indulgence of children

The habit of constantly gratifying every wayward wish and temper under the plea of illness, and the constant indulgence which it meets with in this form from a mother's over-kindness, exert a most injurious influence on the child's character, and it grows up a juvenile hypochondriac.

CHARLES WEST (1816–98)
the founder of the Great Ormond Street Hospital for Sick Children expresses Parkinson's message less poetically

That other inward inbred cause of Melancholy is our temperature, in whole or in part, which we receive from our parents ... Old men beget most part wayward, peevish, sad, melancholy sons, and seldom merry ... Foolish, drunken or hare-brained women most part bring forth children like unto themselves, morose & languid ... if a man eat garlick, onions, fast overmuch, study too hard, be over-sorrowful, dull, heavy, dejected in mind, perplexed in his thoughts, fearful, etc., their sons will be subject to madness & melancholy ... dull, heavy, timorous, discontented, all their lives.

ROBERT BURTON (1577–1640)
The Anatomy of Melancholy

My dear Watson, you as a medical man are continually gaining lights as to the tendencies of a child by the study of the parents. Don't you see that the converse is equally valid? I have frequently gained my first real insight into the character of parents by studying their children.

SIR ARTHUR CONAN DOYLE (1859–1930)
The Adventure of the Copper Beeches

There is no finer investment for any community than putting milk into babies.

SIR WINSTON CHURCHILL (1874–1965)
radio broadcast, 1943

The milk ... the produce of faded cabbage-leaves and sour draff, lowered with hot water, frothed with bruised snails, carried through the streets in open pails, exposed to foul risings discharged from doors and windows, spittle, snot, and tobacco-quids from foot-passengers, over-flowings from mud-carts, spatterings from coach-wheels, dirt and trash chucked into it by roguish boys for joke's sake, the spewing of infants ... and finally, the vermin that drops from the rags of the nasty drab that vends this precious mixture, under the respectable denomination of milk-maid.

TOBIAS SMOLLETT (1721–71)
The Expedition of Humphry Clinker

The literature of disease is more interesting to me than all the healthy books.

T. E. LAWRENCE (1888–1935)

All doctors up to the present century seem to me to have failed, because in the cure of diseases they have given little thought, or none at all, to the specific nature of each disease, and considered only the external symptoms, which are no more concerned with their specific nature than the type and richness of the soil are with species of plants which may grow in it.

> JOHN LOCKE (1632–1704)
> *An Essay Concerning Human Understanding*

The Cramp, the Stitch,
The Squirt, The Itch,
The Gout, the Stone, the Pox;
The Mulligrubs,
The Bonny Scrubs,
And all Pandora's Box.

> AN ADVERTISEMENT OF 'DR' CASE
> seventeenth-century quack

I reckon being ill as one of the greatest pleasures of life, provided one is not too ill and is not obliged to work until one is better.

> SAMUEL BUTLER (1835–1902)
> *The Way of All Flesh*

To be sick is to enjoy monarchal prerogatives.

> CHARLES LAMB (1775–1834)
> *Last Essays of Elia*

It is surprising that the basic sciences single out, for observation and intensive study, phenomena which are most uncommon and hardly of intrinsic significance. Similarly, medicine discusses diseases which are so rare that one does not encounter them more than once or twice during a lifetime with a thoroughness as if the salvation of the art would depend on it.

> JOHANNES DE GORTER (1689–1762)
> *De Motu Vitali*

Common things are common.
ANONYMOUS WARNING AGAINST EXOTIC DIAGNOSIS

In men nine out of ten abdominal tumours are malignant; in women nine out of ten abdominal swellings are the pregnant uterus.
RUTHERFORD MORISON (1853–1939)
The Practitioner, 1965

'Ye can call it influenza if ye like,' said Mrs Machin. 'There was no influence in my young days. We called a cold a cold.'
ARNOLD BENNETT (1867–1931)
The Card

There was one circumstance in particular which distinguished it from ordinary diseases. The birds and animals which feed upon human flesh, although so many bodies were lying unburied, either never came near them, or died if they touched them. This was proved by a remarkable disappearance of the birds of prey, who were not to be seen either about the bodies or anywhere else; while in the case of the dogs the fact was even more obvious, because they live with men.
THUCYDIDES (471–400 BC)
on the plague of Athens 430 BC – probably bubonic plague – from which he recovered

How many good men, how many worthy women, in the prime and vigour of youth – who Galen, Hippocrates or Aesculapius himself would have declared to be in perfect

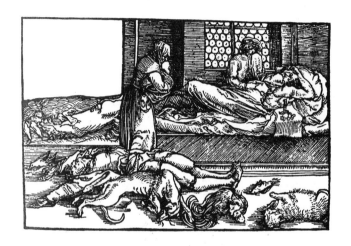

Plague at Augsberg, 1532

health – after dining in the morning with their parents went to sup with their ancestors in the other world?
> GIOVANNI BOCCACCIO (1313–75)
> *The Decameron*
> on the Black Death in Florence

The Tartars, fatigued by such a plague and pestiferous disease, and observing themselves dying without hope of health, ordered the cadavers to be placed on their hurling machines and catapulted into the city of Caffa.
> GABRIEL DE MUSSIS
> on the siege of Caffa in 1346, an early example of bacteriological warfare

Many Persons in the Time of this Visitation never perceiv'd that they were infected, till they found to their unspeakable Suprize, the Tokens come out upon them, after which they seldom liv'd six Hours; for those Spots they call'd the Tokens were really gangreen Spots.
> DANIEL DEFOE (1660–1731)
> *A Journal of the Plague Year*, 1665

Ring-a-ring o' roses,
A pocket full of posies,
Atishoo! Atishoo!
We all fall down.
> NURSERY RHYME
> describing the skin rash produced by the plague,
> herbal attempts to ward off the disease, the initial
> symptoms and ultimate death

To eat is human, to digest divine.
>CHARLES T. COPELAND (1860–1952)

Abstain from beans.
>PYTHAGORAS (sixth century BC)

Flatulence: a collection of gas in the stomach or bowels. In the former case the gas is expelled from time to time in noisy eructations by the mouth; in the latter case it may produce unpleasant rumblings in the bowels, or be expelled from the anus.
>NEWS CHRONICLE HOME DOCTOR, 1931

Was rather uneasy to-day on Account of being afraid that I have got the Piles coming or something else – unless it is owing to my eating a good deal of Peas Pudding two or three days ago with a Leg of Pork.
>JAMES WOODFORDE (1740–1803)
>diary entry for 28 February 1782

Duncan ill with very bad piles – operated on last night, or, since that sounds alarming, lanced. Spoke to Janie of the snobbishness of our sympathies. Cant really sympathize with that particular disease, though the pain is terrible. Must laugh.
>VIRGINIA WOOLF (1882–1941)
>diary entry for 21 July 1934

Had a thorn taken out of the middle of that part of the body which Derham calls a large cushion of flesh by my wife last night.
>BENJAMIN NEWTON
>diary entry for 26 September 1818

Falstaff: What says the doctor to my water?
Page: He said, Sir, the water itself was a good healthy water; but, for the party that owned it, he might have more diseases than he knew for.
WILLIAM SHAKESPEARE (1564–1616)
Henry IV, Part 2

Suddenly yesterday morning I observed that there was bright blood in my pee. Cancer of the bladder, naturally! But I was amazed to find that this assumption hardly seemed to bother me – though I've suffered so cravenly from Timor Mortis all my born days. But when S. consulted one of her medical books it became quite obvious that the culprit was the beetroot we'd had for supper the night before. So my heroic composure was wasted, in a sense, but it's nice to know that I achieved it, however briefly.
PHILIP TOYNBEE (1916–   )
diary entry for 30 December 1978

After I'd written to you yesterday I had an attack of asthma and an incessantly running nose, which forced me to tramp about, lighting cigarettes at every tobacconist etc. And worse was to come: I went to bed about midnight, feeling all right after spending a long time inhaling smoke, but three or four hours later came the real attack of the summer …
MARCEL PROUST (1871–1922)
letter to his mother, 31 August 1901

Female, fat, forty, fecund and filthy.
MEDICAL STEREOTYPE OF PATIENT WITH GALL STONES

I found stones in the ureters, in the bladder, in the colon of the intestine, in the haemorrhoidal veins as well as in the umbilicus. Also in the gall bladder I found stones of various shapes and of various colours.

    MATTEO REALDO COLOMBO
    papal physician, who performed the autopsy on St
    Ignatius Loyola (1491–1556), proving just how
    misleading stereotypes can be

Last night I suffered horribly – from an indigestion ... Query – was it the cockles or what I took to correct them, that caused the commotion? I think both.

    LORD BYRON (1788–1824)
    diary entry for 27 February 1821

I did keep my bed; and my pain continued on me mightily ... but having a good fire in my chamber, I began to break six or seven small and great farts; and so to bed and lay in good ease all night, and pissed pretty well in the morning, but no more wind came as it used to do plentifully, after it once begun, nor any inclination to stool.

    SAMUEL PEPYS (1633–1703)
    diary entry for 7 October 1663

11 April 1681: I took early in the morning, good dose of elixir, and hung three spiders about my neck, and they drove my ague away – *Deo gratias*.

22 May 1682: This night, scratching the right side of my buttock, above the fundament, thence proceeded a violent sharp humour.

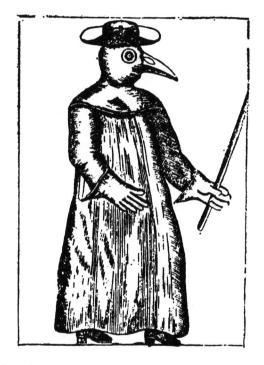

*A plague doctor in Marseilles in 1720 dressed in leather with a snout
filled with purifying spices and a wand to feel pulses at a distance*

4 June 1676: Being hard bound in my body I was five hours before I could go to stool, and suffered much torment.

6 August 1684: I rubbed the skin near my rump, whereupon it began to be very sore.
>   ELIAS ASHMOLE (1617–92)
>   entries from his diary

Half the patients who get you up in the middle of the night and think they are dying are suffering from wind.
>   FRANCIS BRETT YOUNG (1884–1954)
>   *Dr Bradley Remembers*
>   advice to a younger doctor

I woke up early this morning and when I opened the shutters the full round sun was just risen. I began to repeat that verse of Shakespeare's: 'Lo, here the gentle lark weary of rest,' and bounded back into bed. The bound made me cough – I spat – it tasted strange – it was bright red blood – I don't want to find this is real consumption, perhaps it's going to gallop – who knows? – and I shan't have my work written. *That's what matters.* How unbearable it would be to die – leave 'scraps', 'bits' ... nothing real finished.
>   KATHERINE MANSFIELD (1888–1923)
>   diary entry for 19 February 1918

A cough ball of laughter leaped from his throat dragging after it a rattling chain of phlegm.
>   JAMES JOYCE (1882–1941)
>   *Ulysses*, 1922

I would like to remind those responsible for the treatment
of tuberculosis that Keats wrote his best poems while dying
of this disease. In my opinion he would never have done so
under the influence of modern chemotherapy.

ARTHUR WALKER (1896–1955)
Walkerisms

Kept my bed all morning, having laid a poultice to my cods
last night to take down the tumour there which I got
yesterday.

SAMUEL PEPYS (1633–1703)
diary entry for 20 March 1664

Great Venus unmasked, or a more exact discovery of the
venereal evil, or French disease, comprizing the opinions of
the most ancient and modern physicians, with the
particular sentiments of the author touching the rise,
nature, subject, causes, kinds, progress, changes, signs and
prognosticks of the said evil. Together with luculent
problems, pregnant observations, and the most practical
cures of that disease, and virulent gonorrhoea, or running
of the reins. Likewise a tract of general principles of
physick, with discourse of the scurvy, manginess and
plague.

TITLE OF A BOOK BY GIDEON HARVEY (?1640–1700)
physician at the Tower of London. Published 1666

I rose very disconsolate, having rested very ill by the
poisonous infection raging in my veins and anxiety and
vexation boiling in my breast. I could scarcely credit my
own senses. What! thought I. Can this beautiful, this
sensible, and this agreeable woman be so sadly defiled? Can

corruption lodge beneath so fair a form? ... No, it is impossible. I have just got a gleet by irritating the parts too much with excessive venery ... And yet these damned twinges, the scalding heat, and that deep-tinged loathsome matter are the strongest proofs of an infection ... Am I, who have had safe and elegant intrigues with fine women, become the dupe of a strumpet?

> JAMES BOSWELL (1740–95)
> diary entry for 20 January 1763
> a gleet is a discharging lesion caused by gonorrhoea

Lues Boswelliana, or disease of admiration.

> THOMAS BABINGTON MACAULAY (1800–59)
> 'Earl of Chatham': *Essays*

Syphilis has been one of the greatest riddles of the race. For generations it shared with malaria the peculiarity that we knew the cure without knowing the exact cause.

> SIR WILLIAM OSLER (1849–1919), 1909

Here lie two poor Lovers, who had the mishap,
Though very chaste people, to die of a clap.

> ALEXANDER POPE (1688–1744)
> an unkind couplet being an *Epitaph on the Stanton-Harcourt Lovers* who were killed by lightning

Masturbation: the primary sexual activity of mankind. In the nineteenth century it was a disease; in the twentieth it's a cure.

> THOMAS SZASZ (1920–   )
> *The Second Sin*

They are particularly subject to a sidelong gait as though there was a spirit of antagonism set up between the organs of locomotion: one leg being impelled to motion, while the other is strongly impelled to rest.

> DR RUSSELL TRALL
> writing in 1862, on how to identify a masturbating woman by her walk

This abominable Sort of Impurity is that unnatural Practice by which Persons of either Sex may defile their own Bodies, without the Assistance of others, whilst yielding to filthy Imaginations.

> ANONYMOUS AUTHOR OF A TREATISE ON MAS-
> TURBATION
> *Onania or the heinous sin of self-pollution*, 1730

And Onan knew that the seed should not be his ... when he went into his brother's wife that he spilled it on the ground.

> GENESIS 38:9

Because he spills his seed on the ground.

> DOROTHY PARKER (1893–1967)
> when asked why she named her canary 'Onan'

So to my wife's chamber, and there supped and got her cut my hair and look my shirt, for I have itched mightily these six or seven days; and when all came to all, she finds that I am louzy, having found in my head and body above 20 lice, little and great; which I wonder at, being more than I have had I believe almost these 20 years.

> SAMUEL PEPYS (1633–1703)
> diary entry for 23 January 1669

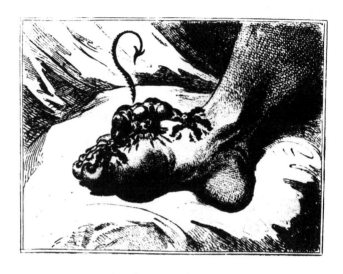

Gout by James Gillray (1799)

The Doctor's Quotation Book

Last Wednesday night while carrying a bucket of water from the well, Hannah Williams slipped upon the icy path and fell heavily upon her back. We fear her spine was injured for though she suffers acute pain in her legs she cannot move them. The poor wild beautiful girl is stopped in her wildness at last, and perhaps by the finger of God.

> FRANCIS KILVERT (1840–79)
> diary entry for 26 December 1874

But only think that during the last six years I have been in a wretched condition, rendered worse by unintelligent physicians. Deceived from year to year with hopes of improvement, and then finally forced to the prospect of lasting infirmity ... Yet it is not possible for me to say to men: speak louder, shout, I am deaf. Alas, how could I declare the weakness of a sense which in me ought to be more acute than in others.

> LUDWIG VAN BEETHOVEN (1770–1827)
> reaction to his deafness, as expressed in his will,
> written in 1802, when he was thirty-two years old

There are two kinds of deafness. One is due to wax and is curable; the other is not due to wax and is not curable.

> SIR WILLIAM WILDE (1815–76)
> ENT surgeon and father of Oscar

There is no paine like the Gowt.

> NICHOLAS BRETON (?1545–?1626)
> *Crossing of Proverbs*

Put your toe in a vice and turn the handle as tight as possible: that is the pain of rheumatism. Give the handle one full turn more: that is the agony of gout.

> ANON

Poor Mr Chute has now had the Gout for these five days with such a degree of pain and uneasiness, as he never felt before. Whether to attribute it to Dr La Cour's forcing medicines, or to a little cold he got as soon as he came hither, I know not, but for above forty hours it seem'd past all human suffering, & he lay screaming like a man on the rack. The torture was so great, that (against my judgement and even his own) he was forced to have recourse to infusion of Poppy-heads.

THOMAS GRAY (1716–71)

Oh! when I have the gout, I feel as if I was walking on my eyeballs.

SYDNEY SMITH (1771–1845)

Smallpox was always present, filling the churchyards with corpses, tormenting with constant fears all whom it had not yet stricken, leaving on those whose lives it spared the hideous traces of its power, turning the babe into a changeling at which the mother shuddered, and making the eyes and cheeks of the betrothed maiden objects of horror to the lover ... She [Queen Mary II] locked herself up during a short time in her closet, burned some papers, arranged others, then calmly awaited her fate.

THOMAS BABINGTON MACAULAY (1800–59)
History of England

Those whom the Gods wish to destroy, they first drive mad.

PROVERB

Everything great in the world comes from neurotics. They alone have founded our religions and composed our masterpieces.

MARCEL PROUST (1871–1922)
Remembrance of Times Past

A mistake which is commonly made about neurotics is to suppose that they are interesting. It is not interesting to be always unhappy, engrossed with oneself, malignant and ungrateful, and never quite in touch with reality.

CYRIL CONNOLLY (1903–74)
The Unquiet Grave

The title I have chosen for this treatise is a reproach universally thrown on this island by foreigners, and all our neighbours on the continent, by whom nervous distempers, spleen, vapours and lowness of spirits are in derision called the English Malady.

GEORGE CHEYNE (1671–1743)
The English Malady

I think for my part one half of the nation is mad – and the other not very sound.

TOBIAS SMOLLETT (1721–71)
The Adventures of Sir Launcelot Greaves

Hamlet: Ay, marry, why was he sent into England?
First Clown: Why, because he was mad; he shall recover his wits there; or, if he do not, 'tis no great matter there.
Hamlet: Why?
First Clown: 'Twill not be seen in him there; there the men are as mad as he.

WILLIAM SHAKESPEARE (1564–1616)
Hamlet

He [King George III] then thus address'd Dr Willis, 'Sir, Your dress and appearance bespeaks You of the Church. Do you belong to it?'

Dr Willis replied, 'I did formerly, but lately I have attended chiefly to physick.'

'I am sorry for it,' answered the King with Emotion and Agitation, 'You have quitted a profession I have always loved, and You have Embraced one I most heartily detest.'

> ROBERT GREVILLE
> diary entry for 5 December 1788 recording 'Mad'
> King George III's reaction to his first meeting with Dr
> Willis, proprietor of a lunatic asylum

Dr Willis had the King confined to his [restraining] Chair this Morning for a short time, and gave Him a severe lecture on his improper conversation, Eliza, &c; His Majesty, becoming more loud and impatient under this Lecture, Dr Willis ordered a Handcherchief to be held before his Mouth, and He then continued and finished his Lecture.

> ROBERT GREVILLE
> diary entry for 30 January 1789

If a patient is poor he is committed to a public hospital as 'psychotic'; if he can afford the luxury of a private sanitarium, he is put there with the diagnosis of 'neurasthenia'; if he is wealthy enough to be isolated in his own home under constant watch of nurses and physicians he is simply an indisposed 'eccentric'.

> PIERRE MARIE JANET (1859–1947)
> *Strength and Psychological Debility*

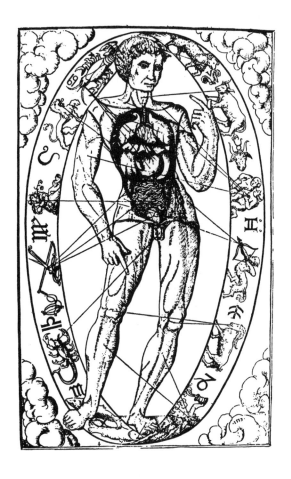

Zodiac man by Jollat (1533)

I am certain now that I am going mad again. It is just as it was the first time, I am always hearing voices ... I have fought against it, but I can't any longer.

VIRGINIA WOOLF (1882–1941)
letter to her sister Vanessa Bell in March 1941,
shortly before she committed suicide

A neuralgic woman seems thus to be peculiarly unfortunate. However bitter and repeated may be her visceral neuralgias, she is either told she is hysterical or that it is all uterus. In the first case she is comparitively fortunate, for she is only slighted; in the second case she is entangled in the net of the gynaecologist, who finds her uterus, like her nose, is a little on the one side, or again, like that organ, is running a little, or it is flabby like her biceps, so that the unhappy viscus is impaled upon a stem, or perched upon a prop, or is painted with carbolic acid every week in the year except during the long vacation when the gynaecologist is grouse-shooting, or salmon-catching, or leading the fashion in the Upper Engadine.

SIR CLIFFORD ALLBUTT (1836–1925)
Lancet, 1884

And with respect to myself, though I have accurately examined my conduct, and scrutinized my soul, I call thee, O God, the searcher of hearts, to witness, that I am not conscious, either in the more early or in the later periods of my life, of having committed any enormity which might deservedly have marked me out as a fit object for such a calamitous visitation.

JOHN MILTON (1608–74)
reaction to his blindness

Those labouring with this Disease [Diabetes], piss a great deal more than they drink ... Authors who affirm the drink to be little or nothing changed are very far from the truth; because the Urine very much differed both from the drink taken in, and also from any humour that is wont to be begot in our Body, [in being] wonderfully sweet as if it were imbued with Honey or Sugar.

> THOMAS WILLIS (1621–75)
> the first to record in modern times the sweet-tasting
> urine found in diabetes ('the pissing evil')
> *Pharmaceutice rationalis*, 1679

'In a case of suspected diabetes, examination of the urine is of paramount importance,' the lecturer told the medical students. 'I want you all to dip your fingers into the sample of urine and taste the sugar.' The doctor demonstrated and each student followed in turn with varying degrees of hesitancy and disgust. 'Medicine is also about the art of appearances,' he continued. 'Notice how I dipped with my index finger and sucked of my ring finger.'

> CAUTIONARY TALE
> of doubtful origin and dubious authenticity

I got my giddiness in 1690 (at the age of 23) by eating 100 golden pippins at a time at Richmond. Four years later at a place 20 miles further on in Surrey I got my deafness; and these two friends have visited me one or other every year since; and being old acquaintances have often sought fit to come together.

> JONATHAN SWIFT (1667–1745)
> describing his Meniere's Disease

I am in the condition of an old fellow of Threescore, with a Complication of Diseases upon me; A constant Headake; ruind Tone of the Stomach; the Piles; a Vomiting & Looseness; & an Excess of Wind. Some of these succeed, the moment I get quit of the others; & upon the whole, indeed I am in a very uncomfortable way.

> ALEXANDER POPE (1688–1744)
> small wonder that these gastric maladies, added to his rickets and spinal tuberculosis, prompted Pope to observe, 'this long disease, my Life' in his *Epistle to Dr Arbuthnot*

A great fit of the stone in my left kidney: all day I could do but three or four drops of water, but I drunk a draught of white wyne and salet oyle, and after that, crabs' eys in powder with the bone in the carp's head, and abowt four of the clok I did eat cake buttered, and with sugar and nutmeg on it, and drunk two great draughts of ale with it; and I voyded within an howr much water and a stone as big as an Alexander seed. God be thanked!

> JOHN DEE (1527–1608)
> diary entry for 31 January 1594

Enter Rheumatism and takes me by the knee. So much for playing the peace-maker in a shower of rain.

> SIR WALTER SCOTT (1771–1832)
> diary entry for 11 January 1827

26 March 1660: This day it is two years since it pleased God that I was cut of the stone at Mrs Turner's in Salisbury Court, and did resolve while I live to keep it a festival.

20 August 1664: I forth to bespeak a case to be made to keep my stone which I was cut of in, which cost me 25s [hillings].

3 May 1667: Thence ... to my Lord Treasurer, who continues still very ill. I had taken my stone with me on purpose, and Sir Philip Warwicke carried it in to him to see, but was not in a condition to talk with me about it, poor man.

    SAMUEL PEPYS (1633–1703)
    three diary entries concerning the stone removed
    from his bladder in 1658

After two days in hospital, I took a turn for the nurse.
    W. C. FIELDS (1879–1945)

For the moment my greatest trouble is the feebleness of my fingers. My pace in writing is that of a child beginning the alphabet. And I am losing the power of spelling.
    CARDINAL NEWMAN (1801–90)
    letter to Dr J. W. Ogle, 12 August 1887

The lives of Type A, coronary-prone, personalities are dominated by time. All is rush. Extreme cases are easily diagnosed as those men who flush the lavatory before they have finished urinating.
    ANON

As men draw near the common goal
Can anything be sadder
Than he who, master of his soul,
Is servant to his bladder?
    ANON
    The Speculum, 1938

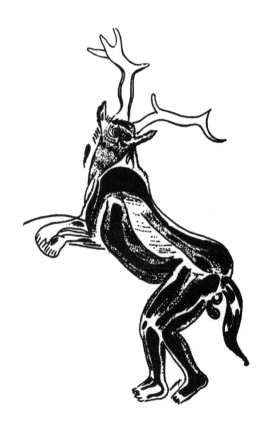

Cro-Magnon medicine man

Similia similibus curantur.
(Similar diseases are cured by similar things.)
>   SAMUEL HAHNEMANN (1755–1843)
>   founder of homoeopathy

When a lot of remedies are suggested for a disease, that means it can't be cured.
>   ANTON CHEKHOV (1860–1904)
>   *The Cherry Orchard*

The remedy is worse than the disease.
>   SIR FRANCIS BACON (1561–1626)
>   'Of Seditions and Troubles': *Essays*

I dressed him, and God healed him.
>   AMBROISE PARÉ (1517–90)
>   *Oeuvres*, 1585

A night with Venus and a lifetime with mercury.
>   TRADITIONAL
>   a reference to the treatment of syphilis with mercurial compounds

Cure for consumption: Cut up a little turf of fresh earth and laying down breathe into the hole a quarter of an hour ... In the last stage suck a healthy woman. This cured my father.
>   JOHN WESLEY (1703–91)
>   *Primitive Physic*

In the year 1775 my opinion was asked concerning a family receipt for the cure of the Dropsy. I was told that it had long been kept a secret by an old woman in Shropshire who had sometimes made cures after the more regular practitioners had failed ... This medicine was composed of twenty or more different herbs; but it was not very difficult for one conversant with these subjects to perceive that the active herb could be no other than the Foxglove.

> WILLIAM WITHERING (1741–99)
> on the use of Foxglove (digitalis) in the treatment of heart disease

He who keeps secret so beneficial an instrument as the harmless obstetrical forceps deserves to have a worm devour his vitals for all eternity.

> DE LA MOTTE
> obstetrician of Volgens. On Hugh Chamberlen's efforts to keep secret details of his obstetric forceps

The people! Could you patent the sun?

> JONAS SALK (1914–   )
> American virologist, when asked who owned the patent on his vaccine for poliomyelitis

If you want a cure for a cold, put on two pullovers, take up a baton, poker or pencil, tune the radio to a symphony concert, stand on a chair, and conduct like mad for an hour or so and the cold will have vanished. It never fails. You know why conductors live so long? Because we perspire so much.

> SIR JOHN BARBIROLLI (1899–1970)
> English conductor

I commenced inhaling the ether before the operation was commenced and continued it until the operation was over. I did not feel the slightest pain from the operation and

could not believe the tumor was removed until it was shown to me.
> JAMES VENABLE
> the first patient to have ether administered in 1842

Who was the man who invented laudanum? I thank him from the bottom of my heart ... I have had six delicious hours of oblivion. Drops, you are darling! If I love nothing else, I love you!
> WILKIE COLLINS (1924–89)
> on his use of laudanum drops, an alcoholic tincture of opium

My heart aches, and a drowsy numbness pains
My sense, as though of hemlock I had drunk,
Or emptied some dull opiate to the drains
One minute past, and Lethe-wards had sunk.
> JOHN KEATS (1795–1821)
> 'Ode to a Nightingale'

Nothing did me any good, but a curious little new fangled operation of putting opium under the skin which relieved one for twenty-four hours – but does not improve the vivacity or serenity of one's intellect.
> FLORENCE NIGHTINGALE (1820–1910)

Sleep only came to her in a red hood of poppies.
> ROBERT BROWNING (1812–89)
> on his wife, Elizabeth Barrett Browning and her addiction to opium and morphia

Woe to you, my Princess, when I come. I will kiss you quite red and feed you till you are plump. And if you are forward, you shall see who is the stronger, a gentle little girl who doesn't eat enough, or a big wild man *who has cocaine in his body*. In my last severe depression I took coca again and a small dose lifted me to the heights in a wonderful fashion. I am now busy collecting the literature for a song of praise to this magical substance.

SIGMUND FREUD (1856–1939)

letter to Martha, his future wife, dated 2 June 1884

When Elisha arrived, he went alone into the room and saw the boy lying dead on the bed. He closed the door and prayed to the Lord. Then he lay down on the boy, placing his mouth, eyes and hands on the boy's mouth, eyes and hands. As he lay stretched out over the boy, the boy's body started to get warm ... The boy sneezed seven times and then opened his eyes.

II KINGS 4: 32–5

scholars are divided whether Elisha's successful resuscitation of the child was due to miraculous intervention or artificial respiration

I leaned forward, opened his mouth and introduced two extended fingers of my right hand as far back as possible, and by pressing the base of his paralysed tongue downward and outward, opened his larynx and made a free passage for air to enter the lungs.

DR CHARLES LEALE

account of his unsuccessful efforts to revive Abraham Lincoln (15 April 1865)

Leeches should be kept a day before applying them. They should be squeezed to make them eject the contents of their stomachs ... The slime and debris should be cleansed from

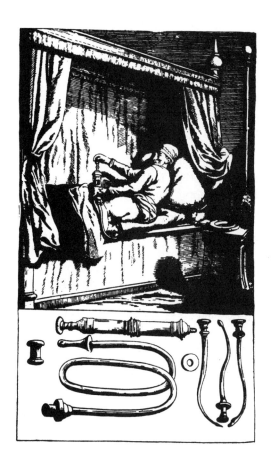

Self administration of an enema using De Graaf's apparatus

their bodies with a sponge … To ensure that they will not crawl into the gullet, nose or anus, one must draw a thread through the tail …

AVICENNA (980–1037)
Arab physician

Cottard, to her [Francoise's] disappointment, gave the preference, though without much hope, to leeches. When, a few hours later, I went into my grandmother's room, fastened to her neck, her temples, her ears, the tiny black reptiles were writhing among her bloodstained locks, as on the head of Medusa.

MARCEL PROUST (1871–1922)
Remembrance of Things Past

On going outside the fort I found an old Pathan graybeard waiting to see me … Eleven days ago he was drinking from a rain-water tank and felt something stick in his throat … I introduced a polypus forceps into the lower part of the pharynx where a body, distinctly moving, was felt … With considerable force I managed to remove it. It was a leech between two-and-a-half and three inches in length with a body of the size of a Lee-Metford bullet. I quote this case as a typical example of the carelessness of natives of the class from which we enlist our Sepoys …

DR GRANGER
surgeon in Her Majesty's Indian Service, writing in
1895, and quoted in Gould and Pyle's *Anomalies and
Curiosities of Medicine*, 1900

At six in the evening, an hour after I had taken my electuary, the tooth-ache returned more violently than ever. I smoked tobacco; which set me vomiting, and took away my senses and pain altogether. At eleven I waked in extreme pain, which I thought would quickly separate soul and body.

CHARLES WESLEY (1816–98)
diary entry for 24 February 1738

From season'd sauce avert your eyes
From hams, and tongues, and pigeon pies.
If ven'son pasty's set before ye,
Each bit you eat memento mori.

GENTLEMAN'S MAGAZINE, 1751
dietary self-help to ward off asthma

Nobles and people of substance keep a sort of little chest supported on four legs like a chair ... A syringe stands up out of the chest like a column ... a tube projects above the box and goes into the anus. In this way the patient can sit on the box as on a horse and insert the piston into the syringe. By pressing with his hand he can easily introduce the fluid into his anus by himself.

BRAMBILLA
Atlas of Surgical Instruments, c. 1780
describing the use of an enema stool

Grace the wyffe of William Baxster, beinge aboute three weekes before her tyme, was brought in bedd the First day of December aboute three of the Clocke in the afternoone of two Children, Their bellies were growne and Joyned together, from their breastes to their Navells, and their faces were together.

JOHN RICHARDSON
seventeenth-century parish clerk near Scarborough,
giving details of Siamese twins, born in 1655

The variety of foreign bodies which have found their way into the rectum is hardly less remarkable than the ingenuity displayed in their removal. A turnip has been delivered per anum by the use of obstetric forceps. A stick firmly impacted has been withdrawn by inserting a gimlet into its lower end. A tumbler, mouth looking downwards, has several times been extracted by filling the interior with a wet plaster of Paris bandage, leaving the end of the bandage extruding, and allowing the plaster to set.

> H. BAILEY AND R. LOVE
> *A Short Practice of Surgery*, 1943

Haslam [1828] records the case of a man who slipped on the greasy deck of a whaler, and falling forward with great violence upon a large knife used to cut blubber, completely severed his penis ... After recovery there was a distinct increase of sexual desire and frequent nocturnal emissions.

There is a record of a tall, powerfully-built Russian peasant of 29, of morose disposition, who on April 3rd [1887], while reading his favourite book, without uttering a cry, suddenly and with a single pull, tore away his scrotum together with his testes. He then arose from the bank where he had been sitting and quietly handed the avulsed parts to his mother. 'Take that. I do not want it anymore.'

> GOULD AND PYLE
> *Anomalies and Curiosities of Medicine*, 1900

On the 13th of June 1812 there occurred an accident which is probably unique in the annals of Medicine. Mr Thomas Tipple, the victim, was unharnessing a horse when the animal lunged and forced the gig-shaft laterally through Tipple's chest. Two farriers found to their astonishment that the shaft had passed through the chest and was protruding several inches on the other side. Tipple was gently pushed towards the end of the shaft thus retracing its path through the thorax. As soon as he was free, and finding his breathing was not affected, he walked into the house.

> FROM WOOD'S MR TIPPLE'S CHEST WOUND
> *Medical History*, July 1960.
> when Tipple died, ten years later, the gig-shaft and anterior chest wall were presented to the Royal College of Surgeons. This prize specimen was destroyed in the blitz in 1941

The contractions of certain muscles enter very importantly into the sexual act. There is a muscular ring, situated at the entrance of the vagina, and known as *constrictor cunni*. In some women this ring contracts in sexual excitement. It seizes the male member, so to speak, and draws it deep into the vagina ... However these muscular movements are rather rare in civilized women, and the *constrictor cunni* appears to be in course of retrogression.

> WILLY, VANDER AND FISHER
> *Encyclopaedia of Sex Practice*, 1933

It is by ... accurate observations in Practice that we must improve our Knowledge in the State of Physic and Disease; it is this Knowledge, and these Abilitys, that must be the distinguishing *Characteristic* of a true *Physician*, from an Empiric; it is from this method of reasoning from Data, founded upon Observations and real facts, that the *Healing Art* must be improved and brought to a State of Perfection.

> WILLIAM HILLARY (–1763)
> part of the preface of A *Rational and Mechanical Essay on the Small Pox*, 1735

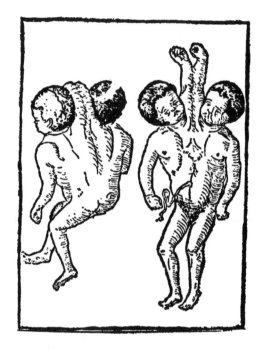

Siamese twins born in Landshut, 1517

Thus I saw that most men only care for science so far as they get a living by it, and that they worship even error when it affords them a subsistence.
JOHANN VON GOETHE (1749–1832)

The body is but a pair of pincers set over a bellows and a stewpan and the whole fixed upon stilts.
SAMUEL BUTLER (1835–1902)
Note-Books

When I first gave my mind to vivisection, as a means of discovering the motions and uses of the heart, and sought to discover these from actual inspection, and not from the writings of others, I found the task so truly arduous, so full of difficulties, that I was almost tempted to think with Fracastorius, that the motion of the heart was only to be comprehended by God.
WILLIAM HARVEY (1578–1657)
On the Motion of the Heart and Blood in Animals

I'll rediscover my disease: I know it exists; I feel it; and I'll prove it if I have to experiment on every mortal animal that got a liver at all.
GEORGE BERNARD SHAW (1856–1950)
The Philanderer
Dr Paramore railing against vivisectional constraints

There are people who do not object to eating a mutton chop – people who do not even object to shooting a pheasant with the considerable chance that it may be only wounded and may have to die after lingering in pain, unable to obtain its proper nutriment – and yet who consider it something monstrous to introduce under the skin of a guinea pig a little inoculation of some microbe to ascertain its action. These seem to me to be most inconsistent views.

> LORD LISTER (1827–1912)
> writing in the *British Medical Journal*, 1897

I injected wine and ale into the mass of blood in a living dog, by a vein, in good quantities, till he became extremely drunk … It will be too long to tell you the effects of opium, scammony and other things which I have tried in this way.

> SIR CHRISTOPHER WREN (1632–1723)
> architect and inventor of intravenous drug adminis-
> tration, describing his techniques to Sir William
> Petty

I know not that by living dissections any discovery has been made by which a single malady is more easily cured.

> SAMUEL JOHNSON (1709–84)
> *The Idler*, 1758

I would rather that any white rabbit on earth should have Asiatic cholera twice than that I should have it just once.

> IRVIN S. COBB (1876–1944)

Many persons nowadays seem to think that any conclusion must be very scientific if the arguments in favor of it are derived from twitching of frogs' legs – especially if the frogs are decapitated – and that – on the other hand – any doctrine chiefly vouched for by the feelings of human beings – with heads on their shoulders – must be benighted and superstitious.

> WILLIAM JAMES (1842–1910)
> *Pragmatism*

The great tragedy of Science: the slaying of a beautiful hypothesis by an ugly fact.
>THOMAS HUXLEY (1825–95)
>*Biogenesis and Abigenesis*

False facts are highly injurious to the progress of science, for they often endure long; but false views, if supported by some evidence, do little harm, for every one takes salutary pleasure proving their falseness.
>CHARLES DARWIN (1809–92)
>*The Descent of Man, and Selection in Relation to Sex*, 1871

A spectre haunts our culture. It is that people will eventually be unable to say 'We fell in love and married' ... but will, as a matter of course, say, 'Our libidinal impulses being reciprocal, we integrated our individual erotic drives and brought them within the same frame of reference.'
>SIR ERNEST GOWERS' OSLERIAN ORATION
>*Medical Jargon*, 1958, in which he quotes Lionel Trilling

I know there are professors in this country who 'ligate' arteries. Other surgeons only tie them, and it stops the bleeding just as well.
>OLIVER WENDELL HOLMES (1809–94)
>*Medical Essays*

Gottimhimmelpekker: penis envy
>AN ILLUSTRATION OF A PSYCHIATRIST'S PENCHANT
>FOR GERMAN JARGON

It is most certainly to you that I owe Sherlock Holmes, and although in the stories I have the advantage of being able to place him in all sorts of dramatic situations, I do not think that his analytical work is in the least exaggeration of some effects which I have seen you produce in the out-patient ward.

SIR ARTHUR CONAN DOYLE (1859–1930)
writing in 1892 to Dr Joseph Bell, his inspiration for Sherlock Holmes

I knew myself at the first breath of this new life to be more wicked, tenfold more wicked … and the thought in that moment braced and delighted me like wine.

ROBERT LOUIS STEVENSON
The Strange Case of Dr Jekyll and Mr Hyde, 1886
description of the change which came over Dr Jekyll

For two years, each day, Beaumont tied pieces of meat, potatoes, bread, fruit and vegetables to a silk string, and these he lowered into the wound … He would withdraw these tasties at varying intervals, to record in his notebook the exact state of the particle's decomposition.

RICHARD SELZER (1928–   )
Mortal Lessons
describing the debt that William Beaumont extracted from Alexis St Martin after Beaumont had helped him survive a stomach wound which left him with a permanent fistula, 1822

Don't come for autopsy. Will be killed.

warning telegram to Sir William Osler not to claim the stomach of Alexis St Martin at his death in 1880, aged 86 years.

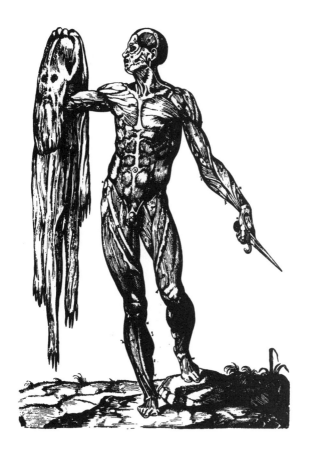

By de Hamusco (1556)

In the years 1813–14, when Mr Astley Cooper was rising towards his zenith, and when Bright was a medical neophyte fresh from Cambridge, there lived in the Borough as students of Guy's and St Thomas's, three young men, who occupied the same rooms, and who seem to have enjoyed their lives as only men in the spring of life can. Their names were John Keats, Henry Stephens and George Wilson Mackereth ... Here, one evening in the twilight, the students sitting together, Stephens at his medical studies, Keats at his dreaming, Keats broke out to Stephens that he had composed a new line:

A thing of beauty is a constant joy

'What do you think of that, Stephens?'
'It has a true ring but is wanting in some way,' replies the latter, as he dips once more into his medical studies. An interval of silence, and again the poet:

A thing of beauty is a joy for ever

'What do you think of that Stephens?'
'That will live for ever.'
BENJAMIN WARD RICHARDSON
The Asclepiad, January 1884

Men are not going to embrace eugenics. They are going to embrace the first likely, trim-figured girl with limpid eyes and flashing teeth who comes along, in spite of the fact that her germ plasm is probably reeking with hypertension, cancer, haemophilia, colour blindness, hay fever, epilepsy, and amyotrophic lateral sclerosis.
LOGAN CLENDENING (1884–1945)

Price, William, VSLM. Llantrissant. MRCS Eng. & LSA. 1821 (St. Barthol. & Lond. Hosp.). Decipherer of 'Gwyllllis yn Nayd'. Discoverer of Gavval Lenn Berren Myrdhdhin Wyllt Tyurn wialenn Oyurr Aneurin Gwawtrudh Awennudh Privv Varrydh Nuadh y Brunn Gwunn Gwialen Lann ab Lann ab Beyl ap Peyl Sarrph ynus Pruttann A ych Choyul Brenn Privv Varrydh Duscc Cymmru a Gwyllllis yn Nayd.

> MEDICAL DIRECTORY 1886
> the entry in the *Medical Directory* of 1886 for William
> Price, doctor, schizophrenic, writer of unintelligible
> Welsh and pioneer of cremation when he partially
> incinerated his dead baby son, Jesus Christ Price, in
> Llantrisant in 1884

The Membranous Envelope [a condom] is prepared from the bladder of a fish caught in the Rhine. Its extreme thinness does not in the least interfere with the pleasure of the act … [its use] is of the greatest utility because, while it is a sure preventive of contraception, it also prevents either party from contracting disease.

> EDWARD BLISS FOOTE
> *Medical Common Sense*, 1864
> a pioneering advocate of birth control

Flashed through the land the electric message came:
He is not better; he is much the same.

> ANONYMOUS WIT
> the daily medical bulletins about the Prince of Wales,
> signed by William Jenner and William Gull, were
> relayed world-wide on the newly invented electric
> telegraph, 1871

This is the house of full and plenty –
You come in full, and you go out empty.
> ANON
> description of a Dublin maternity hospital. A
> reference both to the pregnant patients and the
> students' crates of stout

I can think of no better step to signalize the inauguration of the National Health Service than that a person who so obviously needs psychiatric attention should be among the first of its patients.
> SIR WINSTON CHURCHILL (1874–1965)
> speaking in 1948, about Aneurin Bevan, founder of
> the NHS

The change of the underwear is a refinement that is not commonly practiced, but it adds much, indeed, to the after-comfort of the surgeon, and not a little to his personal safety in the instances of tedious effort in a hot room.
> JOSEPH BRYANT
> *Operative Surgery*, 1900

Authors, you know, of greatest Fame
Thro' Modesty supress their Name;
And wou'd you wish me to reveal,
What these superior Wits conceal? ...

All my Ambition is, I own,
To profit and to please, unknown.
> NATHANIEL COTTON (1705–88)
> *Visions in Verse for the Entertainment and Instruction of*
> *Younger Minds*
> justifiable modesty of this physician and one-time
> psychiatrist of Cowper

Visitors are no proper companions in the chamber of sickness. They come when I could sleep or read, they force me to attend when my mind calls for relaxation, and to speak when my powers will hardly actuate my tongue.

    SAMUEL JOHNSON (1709–84)
    letter dated 27 December 1783

The ultimate indignity is to be given a bedpan by a stranger who calls you by your first name.

    MAGGIE KUHN (1905–   )
    The Observer, 1978

That should assure us of at least 45 minutes of undisturbed privacy.

    DOROTHY PARKER (1893–1967)
    The Algonquin Wits
    on pressing a bell for a nurse

Ambulance: a vehicle for conveying stretchers upon which sick or wounded persons are laid for removal.

    NEWS CHRONICLE HOME DOCTOR, 1931

Norik Hakpioan, 24, was found naked with 90% burns. The fumes from an open bottle of petrol had been ignited by a cooker hotplate. His brother told the coroner that relieving piles with paraffin was an old family remedy and that possibly Norik had mistaken petrol for paraffin.

    AFTER THE DAILY TELEGRAPH, 6 October 1982

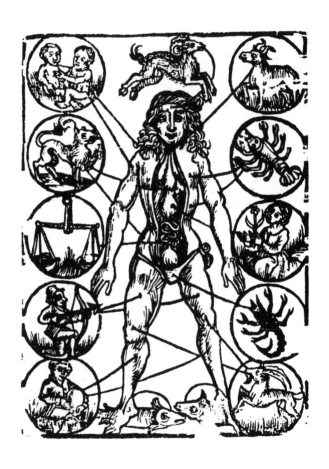

By de'Luzzi (1316)

'You are old, father William,'
The young man cried,
'The few locks which are left you are grey;
You are hale, father William,
A hearty old man;
Now tell me the reason I pray.'
    ROBERT SOUTHEY (1774–1843)
    'The Old Man's Comforts and How He Gained
    Them.'

'In my youth,' said the sage,
As he shook his grey locks,
'I kept all my limbs very supple
By the use of this ointment –
One shilling the box –
Allow me to sell you a couple?'
    LEWIS CARROLL (1832–98)
    Alice in Wonderland

Forty years on, growing older and older,
Shorter in wind and in memory long,
Feeble of foot and rheumatic of shoulder,
What will it help you that once you were young?
    HARROW SCHOOL SONG

There are two things which Man cannot look at directly
without flinching: the sun and death.
    DUC FRANCOIS DE LA ROCHEFOUCAULD (1613–80)
    Maxims

Dream that my little baby came to life again; that it had only been cold, and that we rubbed it before the fire, and it lived. Awake and find no baby.
    MARY SHELLEY (1797–1851)
    diary entry for 19 March 1815

Senescence begins
And middle age ends,
The day your descendants
Outnumber your friends.
    OGDEN NASH (1902–71)

Longevity: Uncommon extension of the fear of death.
    AMBROSE BIERCE (1842–1914)
    The Devil's Dictionary

No young man believes he shall ever die.
    WILLIAM HAZLITT (1778–1830)
    The Monthly Magazine, 1827

Body and mind, like man and wife, do not always agree to die together.
    CHARLES C. COLTON (?1780–1832)
    Lacon

The first sign of his approaching end was when my old aunts, while undressing him, removed a toe with one of his socks.
    GRAHAM GREENE (1904–91)
    Travels With My Aunt

Last scene of all,
That ends this strange eventful history,
Is second childishness, and mere oblivion,
Sans teeth, sans eyes, sans taste, sans everything.
>   WILLIAM SHAKESPEARE (1564–1616)
>   *As You Like It*

Objectionable people are numerous. They have one trait in common, that is, a most unfortunate tendency to longevity.
>   J. CHALMERS DA COSTA (1863–1933)
>   *Selected Papers and Speeches*

Most philosophers, most great men, most anatomists, and most other men of eminence lie like the devil.
>   WILLIAM HUNTER (1718–83)
>   Male midwife and anatomist

If I had the strength to hold a pen, I would write how easy and pleasant a thing it is to die.
>   WILLIAM HUNTER (1718–83)

It is the duty of a doctor to prolong life. It is not his duty to prolong the act of dying.
>   LORD THOMAS HORDER (1871–1955)
>   speech in House of Lords, 1936

If they get into the habit of doing such a thing [euthanasia] when a person is in a hopeless state, why, they *may* do it when a person is *not* in a hopeless state.
>   WILLIAM LAMB, LORD MELBOURNE (1779–1848)
>   quoted by Queen Victoria in her diary, 1838

The heroin in her system might have killed her immediately. It did not. When, after a while, she walked out to the lobby, she could not have known she was dying. There she chatted with the hotel clerk for a second and asked him to change a five-dollar bill for cigarettes, which she purchased. Then she went back to her room. Closing the door, she stepped forward a foot or two and fell, like a puppet hurled down or kicked over.

MYRA FRIEDMAN's biography of blues singer, Janis Joplin (1943–1970)
Buried Alive

The reports of my death are greatly exaggerated.

MARK TWAIN (1835–1910)
cable from Europe to Associated Press

'Mon Dieu! What are you looking at? How can you stare like that? You look like a calf that has just had its throat cut.'

GEORGE II (1683–1760)
to his wife Queen Caroline as she lay dying.

When the news of Napoleon's death came, before the King had been informed of it by his Ministers, Sir E. Nagle, anxious to communicate the welcome tidings, said to him, 'Sir, your bitterest enemy is dead.'

'Is she, by God!' said the tender husband.

HENRY EDWARD FOX
diary entry for 25 August 1821

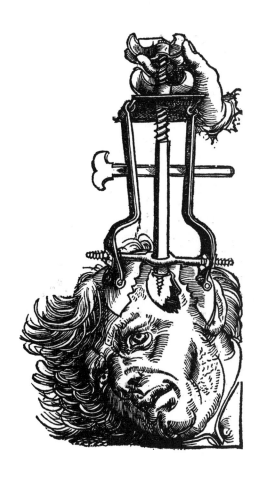

Apparatus for depressed fractures

Any man's death diminishes me, because I am involved in
Mankinde;
And therefore never send to know for whom the bell tolls;
It tolls for thee.

  JOHN DONNE (1573–1631)
  Devotions

 For there is good news yet to hear and fine things to be
  seen,
Before we go to Paradise by way of Kensal Green.
  G.K. CHESTERTON (1874–1936)
  'Before the Roman Came to Rye'

Here lies a poor woman, who always was tired;
She lived in a house where help was not hired.
Her last words on earth were: 'Dear friends I am going
Where washing ain't done, nor sweeping, nor sewing;
But everything there is exact to my wishes;
For where they don't eat there's no washing of dishes …

Don't mourn for me now; don't mourn for me never –
I'm going to do nothing for ever and ever.
  ANON
  The Tired Woman's Epitaph, written before 1850